The Obesity Cure Diet

A Strategy For Overcoming Appetite Urges, Reduce Weight and Increase Vitality

By

Jaden Chapman

Disclaimer
Copyright © 2024 by Jaden Chapman.

The Obesity Cure

Table of contents

Introduction

Implications of the obesity pandemic

The term "obesity epidemic" describes a marked and pervasive rise in the prevalence of obesity in a population. It is typified by a high percentage of overweight or obese individuals, which frequently results in several health problems like diabetes, heart disease, and other related illnesses.

The obesity epidemic has broad ramifications that touch on many different areas. They are as follows:

Health consequences

One of the main risk factors for conditions like heart disease, type 2 diabetes, and some cancers is obesity.

Diabetes Type 2

Cells that are obese frequently develop insulin resistance, which reduces their insulin sensitivity. Type 2 diabetes may develop as a result of high blood sugar levels.

Consequences

Diabetes that is not managed over an extended period can cause consequences like nerve damage, kidney damage, and cardiovascular disease.

Consequences

Obesity increases the risk of heart conditions such as coronary artery disease, heart attacks, and heart failure.

Excessive blood pressure, or hypertension

Because the body needs more blood to support its growing amount of fat tissue, blood volume increases and arterial wall pressure rises.

Consequences

Chronically high blood pressure increases the risk of cardiovascular events by putting strain on the heart and arteries.

Some Cancers

Certain cancers, such as kidney, endometrial, breast, and colorectal cancers, are more likely to occur in obese people.

Heart-related Conditions

High blood pressure and atherosclerosis, or the hardening of the arteries, are two conditions that are exacerbated by obesity. The risk of heart disease and stroke is raised by these variables.

Repercussions

The precise mechanisms are multifaceted and encompass alterations in hormone levels, inflammation, and insulin resistance.

Apnea in Sleep

Breathing disruptions during sleep can result from airway narrowing brought on by excess body weight, particularly in the vicinity of the neck.

As a result, sleep apnea has been connected to a higher risk of cardiovascular problems, daytime fatigue, and other health issues.

Non- Alcoholic Fatty Liver Disease(NAFLD)

Fat buildup in the liver due to obesity can result in non-alcoholic fatty liver disease (NAFLD), which damages and inflames the liver.

As a result, NAFLD may lead to more serious diseases such as cirrhosis and non-alcoholic steatohepatitis (NASH).

Joint Osteoarthritis

Being overweight puts extra strain on joints that support weight, which causes cartilage to deteriorate. Osteoarthritis is largely predisposed to obesity, especially in the knees and hips.

Stroke

Hypertension and atherosclerosis are linked to obesity and raise the risk of blood clots and blockages in blood vessels that supply the brain.

Increased risk of strokes, which have the potential to seriously harm the nervous system, is the result.

Implications On The Social and Psychological Levels

Stigma and Discrimination

Individuals who are obese frequently experience bias and discrimination, which can worsen mental health problems, cause social isolation, and lower self-esteem. Unfavorable body image stereotypes could be a part of the societal prejudice that surrounds obese people.

Mental Health

Mental health issues like anxiety and depression are associated with obesity. An individual's mental health may be impacted by pressure from society to meet physical standards and by having a negative body image.

Effect on Interpersonal Relationships

People who are obese may find it difficult to establish and sustain relationships because of prejudices and preconceived notions held by society. Friendships, romantic relationships, and social interactions may all be impacted by this.

Quality of life

The quality of life can be negatively impacted by obesity by preventing one from engaging in some social and recreational activities. This limitation may exacerbate feelings of alienation and annoyance.

Adaptive Techniques

There is a cycle of weight gain and emotional distress when people turn to food as a coping mechanism for emotional stress. This may also exacerbate psychological issues.

Chapter 1

What Is the Obesity Epidemic's Primary Cause?

Numerous variables, mainly related to diet, can be attributed to the development of the obesity pandemic, including:

Low-Nutritional-Value, High-Calorie Foods

Foods that are high in energy (calories) but lacking in important vitamins, minerals, and other nutrients are referred to as high-calorie, low-nutrient foods.

Among the traits are:

High Energy

These foods include a lot of calories, which is frequently because they are high in refined carbohydrates, harmful fats, or sugar.

Insufficient in Nutrients

These foods are high in calories but lacking in vital elements like antioxidants, fiber, vitamins, and minerals.

Unsatisfactory Contentment

Eating foods high in calories but poor in nutrients may not make you feel full or satiated, which could lead to overeating.

Here are some examples of high-calorie and low-nutrient foods;
Items from Fast Food Restaurants
Many fast food choices are well-known for being high in calories while being low in nutrients. Burgers, fries, and sugary beverages are all examples.

Snacks That Have Been Processed
Chips, cookies, candies, and other processed snacks frequently contain added sugars, bad fats, and little or no nutritional value.

Beverages with Added Sugar

Sugary drinks, such as sodas, energy drinks, and sweetened fruit juices, contain a lot of calories but no essential nutrients.

Specific Baked Goods

 Pastries, cakes, and other baked goods frequently have high levels of sugar and unhealthy fats, which contribute to their energy density.

Foods for Convenience

Pre-packaged meals, microwaveable dinners, and certain convenience foods can contain a lot of calories.

Sedentary Lifestyle

Because of desk jobs, increased screen time, and reliance on transportation for even short distances, modern lifestyles frequently involve less physical activity. Sedentary behavior causes a discrepancy between calorie intake and expenditure, which in turn leads to a decrease in physical activity and the obesity epidemic. The absence of regular exercise raises the risk of obesity-related health issues, decreases metabolism, and encourages weight gain. Long periods of sitting can also have a detrimental effect on insulin sensitivity and metabolic health, which increases the risk of weight gain.

High-Fat Diets

Diets high in saturated and trans fats, which are commonly found in fried foods, processed snacks, and certain oils, can contribute to weight gain and hurt cardiovascular health.

Fast Food Culture

The prevalence of fast-food culture, which is characterized by readily available, high-calorie, and often unhealthy food options, can contribute to poor dietary choices.

Promotion of Unhealthy Foods

Aggressive marketing of sugary and high-calorie foods, particularly to children, can influence consumer choices and contribute to overconsumption.

Lack of Education

Inadequate nutrition and healthy eating education can lead to poor dietary choices, with individuals unaware of the impact of their food choices on overall health.

Medication and Treatment

Certain medications and medical treatments may cause weight gain as a side effect.

Socioeconomic Factors

Due to financial constraints, limited access to healthy foods can lead to a reliance on cheaper, processed alternatives.

Lower levels of education may also be associated with a lack of awareness of healthy lifestyle options.

Psychological Factors
Stress and Emotional Eating

Stressful lifestyles and emotional factors may cause overeating as a coping mechanism. Stress and emotional eating, which frequently result in overeating, particularly of comfort foods and high-calorie items, are contributing factors to the obesity pandemic. The hormone cortisol, which is released by the body in stressful circumstances, can cause cravings for fatty and sugary foods. Emotional eating can lead to overindulgence in calories since it is motivated by emotions rather than hunger. These actions could develop into habits over time and lead to weight gain and obesity.

Furthermore, emotional eating can obstruct the body's normal signals of hunger and fullness, making it difficult to maintain a healthy weight.

Chapter 2

The Hormonal Basis of Obesity.

The hormones that control hunger, metabolism, and energy balance are all involved in the complex hormonal mechanisms of obesity. The following provides a thorough explanation of several important hormones anhow obesity develops as a result of them:

Leptin

Leptin is a hormone that is mostly produced by adipocytes, or fat cells, and it is essential for controlling body weight and energy balance. Its main purpose is to transmit information about the body's stored fat content to the brain, specifically the hypothalamus.

Mechanism of Regulation of Appetite

As a satiety signal, leptin informs the brain that there is no need to eat more because the body already has enough energy stored. Thus, it aids in controlling appetite.

Resistance to Leptin

Leptin resistance is a paradoxical condition that frequently arises in obesity. The brain becomes less receptive to leptin's signals even at elevated levels. Because of this decreased sensitivity, even in situations where the body has an abundance of stored fat, the brain may believe that the body is experiencing a relative energy deficit.

Ghrelin

Ghrelin is sometimes referred to as the "hunger hormone" due to its ability to increase appetite and encourage food consumption. It acts on the brain's hypothalamus and is mostly produced in the stomach.

Mechanism
Stimulation of Appetite

Before meals, ghrelin levels usually increase, alerting the brain that the body needs food. The increase in ghrelin is one factor that causes hunger.

Meal Commencement

The start of a meal is signaled by the release of ghrelin, and its levels drop after consumption.

Hormonal Imbalance and Modified Regulation in Obesity

There may be abnormalities in the normal regulation of ghrelin in obese individuals. This may result in abnormal appetite patterns and possibly insufficient hunger cues.

Overeating

Overeating can lead to weight gain if there is insufficient post-meal suppression or elevated ghrelin levels.

Preference for Foods High in Energy
Dysregulation of ghrelin may affect one's appetite and cause one to favor foods high in energy and frequently unhealthy.

Insulin
The main function of the hormone insulin, which is produced by the pancreas, is to control the body's levels of glucose, or blood sugar. It makes it easier for cells, particularly muscle and fat cells, to absorb glucose for storage or energy.

Mechanism of Regulation of Glucose

The pancreas releases insulin when blood sugar levels rise after a meal. Insulin lowers blood sugar levels by facilitating cells' absorption of glucose from the bloodstream.

Keeping Extra Energy Stored

Extra glucose is encouraged to be converted into glycogen by insulin so that it can be temporarily stored in the muscles and liver. Excess glucose is transformed into fat and stored for a long time in adipose tissue when these storage capacities are filled.

Insulin Resistance

This is the state in which cells lose their sensitivity to the actions of insulin. This implies that to maintain normal blood sugar levels, higher insulin levels are required.

Relationship with Obesity

Insulin resistance is closely linked to obesity, especially when extra fat builds up around the abdominal organs.

Insulin Resistance's Effects

Increased Fat Storage

Weight gain, particularly in the abdominal region, can be attributed to insulin resistance because it can promote more effective fat storage.

Metabolic Syndrome Risk

One of the main elements of metabolic syndrome, which is a collection of disorders that includes high blood pressure, elevated blood sugar, and abnormal cholesterol levels, is insulin resistance.

Elements That Lead to Insulin Resistance

Being Overweight

Substances released by excess adipose tissue, especially visceral fat, can disrupt the functions of insulin.

Lack of Exercise

Insulin resistance is linked to inactivity regularly.

Poor Eating Habits

Insulin resistance may be exacerbated by diets heavy in unhealthy fats and refined carbohydrates.

The Hormone Estrogen.

A class of hormones known as estrogen is vital to the growth and operation of the female reproductive system.

Estrogen affects many physiological processes, such as metabolism and fat distribution, in addition to its reproductive roles.

Mechanism

Fat Distribution

The distribution of body fat is significantly influenced by estrogen. Estrogen tends to encourage subcutaneous fat storage in premenopausal women as opposed to visceral fat storage around organs.

The Metabolic process

By increasing insulin sensitivity, estrogen affects metabolism and may lower the risk of insulin resistance and type 2 diabetes.

Regulation of Appetite

In addition to regulating appetite, estrogen also affects hunger and food intake, and its levels can fluctuate during the menstrual cycle.

Changes in Hormones During Menopause

The menopause causes a decrease in estrogen levels. Changes in the distribution of fat, including an increase in abdominal fat, are linked to this hormonal shift.

Impact on Metabolism

A lower metabolic rate and a higher chance of developing insulin resistance are associated with a decrease in estrogen.

Applicability to Obesity
Obesity Risk and Estrogen

Reduced estrogen levels, which are common in menopause and other hormonally imbalanced conditions, may raise the risk of obesity.

Impact on Fat Cell Function Estrogen has an impact on fat cells' size, composition, and capacity to store and release energy.

Cortisol

The steroid hormone cortisol, which is produced by the adrenal glands, is vital to the body's response to stress. It is frequently referred to as the "stress hormone."In addition to its role in the stress response, cortisol is involved in other physiological systems, including metabolism, the immune system, and blood pressure regulation.

Stress Reaction Mechanism

Cortisol is released in response to psychological or physical stress. By increasing blood sugar and releasing stored energy, it gets the body ready for the "fight or flight" reaction.

The Process of Metabolization

Cortisol influences metabolism by boosting the amount of glucose that may be used as fuel by promoting the breakdown of proteins into amino acids.

Defense Mechanism

Because cortisol has anti-inflammatory qualities, it aids the body in regulating inflammation when under stress.

Dysregulation of Cortisol in Obesity

Persistent elevation of cortisol levels can result from chronic stress, both psychological and physical, and can aggravate metabolic disorders.

Resistance to Cortisol

A type of cortisol resistance, in which the body's tissues lose sensitivity to the hormone's effects, may exist in certain obese individuals.

Effects of an Unbalanced Cortisol Level

Insulin resistance is linked to prolonged elevations in cortisol levels, and this can lead to weight gain and a higher risk of type 2 diabetes.

Sleep Disturbance

There is a circadian rhythm to cortisol levels; they are higher in the morning and lower in the evening. Sleep disturbances can be caused by disruptions in this rhythm, which are frequently observed in chronic stress.

Reduced Immune Response

Prolonged high cortisol levels can weaken the immune system and make a person more vulnerable to infections.

Chapter 3

How Sugar Affects Obesity and Stomach Fat Deposition

When you consume sugar, especially in the form of refined sugars and high-fructose corn syrup, it rapidly boosts blood glucose levels. Insulin, a hormone that aids cells in absorbing glucose for energy, is released in response to this. On the other hand, consuming too much sugar might cause insulin resistance, a condition in which cells are unable to react to insulin as well.

Overindulging in sugar consumption can result in weight gain and fat deposition, especially around the abdomen. Consuming a lot of sugar raises insulin levels, which encourages fat storage. Additionally, sweet foods generally lack nutritional value, resulting in overeating and a calorie excess, which can lead to obesity over time.

Insulin resistance has a role in obesity and the accumulation of fat around the stomach through a number of interrelated pathways.

Elevated Insulin Levels

In order to control blood sugar, insulin resistance requires elevated insulin levels. Increased insulin encourages fat storage, particularly in fat cells found in the abdomen.

Improved Fat Retention

Adipose tissue stores glucose as fat when insulin levels are high. Insulin-resistant cells convert more glucose into fat because they are less able to store glucose as glycogen in muscles.

Encouragement of Lipogenesis

Insulin resistance encourages the body to produce more fatty acids from glucose through a process called lipogenesis. The accumulation of fat is facilitated by the storage of these fatty acids in fat cells.

Storage of Fat in the Abdomen

The type of fat linked to insulin resistance, known as visceral fat, typically gathers in the abdominal region. Visceral fat has a higher metabolic activity and is associated with an increased risk of obesity-related health issues.

Effect on Regulation of Appetite

Increased desires and excessive calorie consumption may result from insulin resistance's disruption of the appetite-regulating system. The excess of calories that result adds to the total weight gain.

Inflammatory Factors

Chronic low-grade inflammation is promoted by insulin resistance and the obesity that goes along with it. Insulin resistance has a role in the release of inflammatory chemicals. Inflammation can aggravate the buildup of fat and further interfere with metabolic functions.

Imbalances in hormones

Insulin interacts with ghrelin and leptin, two additional hormones involved in metabolism.

The balance of these hormones can be upset by insulin resistance, which can affect signals of hunger and satiety.

Due to inadequate satiety signals, blood sugar swings, and their relationship with emotional and thoughtless eating, sugary foods' lack of nutritional value might cause overeating. This pattern accumulates fat over time, especially around the abdomen, and leads to obesity. A healthy weight can be maintained and related health problems can be avoided by selecting meals that are high in nutrients and well-balanced.

In conclusion, insulin resistance stimulates greater fat storage, interferes with appetite regulation, and contributes to a pro-inflammatory state, all of which are critical factors in the development of obesity and fat accumulation around the stomach. In order to control weight and minimize related health concerns, it is imperative to address insulin resistance by lifestyle modifications such as eating a balanced diet and getting regular exercise.

Chapter 4

Fats that Make You Gain Weight and Fats That Make You Lose Weight

Your body composition is influenced by the type of fats you consume. Weight gain can be exacerbated by saturated and trans fats, which are commonly found in processed foods. Unsaturated fats, such as those found in avocados and nuts, on the other hand, can be part of a healthy diet and may aid in weight management when consumed in moderation.

Fats That Cause Weight Gain
Saturated Fatty Acid

Saturated fats are fats in which the carbon atoms are completely saturated with hydrogen atoms, implying that there are no double bonds between the carbon atoms. At normal room temperature, they typically exist in a solid state.

Saturated fats are primarily found in animal-based products such as red meat, full-fat dairy (whole milk, cheese, butter), skin-on poultry, and certain tropical oils such as coconut oil and palm oil.

Effect on Weight

A high intake of saturated fats can lead to weight gain and obesity. These fats are high in energy and, if not consumed in moderation, can lead to an excess of calories.

Health Impact of Saturated fats

Saturated fat-rich diets have been linked to an increased risk of cardiovascular disease. High intake is linked to higher levels of LDL (low-density lipoprotein) cholesterol, also known as "bad" cholesterol. This can contribute to plaque buildup in arteries, which can lead to atherosclerosis and an increased risk of heart disease.

Recommendations

Saturated fat consumption should be limited and replaced with healthier alternatives such as unsaturated fats, according to health guidelines. This can be accomplished by using leaner cuts of meat, low-fat or fat-free dairy products, and healthier cooking oils.

Trans Fats

Trans fats, also known as trans fatty acids, are unsaturated fats with an unusual chemical structure. They are made through a process known as hydrogenation, in which hydrogen is added to liquid vegetable oils to solidify them. Some naturally occurring unsaturated fatty acids are converted into trans-unsaturated fatty acids during this process.

Trans fats are classified into two types:

Trans Fats Found in Nature
These are found in trace amounts in animal products such as meat and dairy. The primary concern, however, is with industrially produced trans fats.

Trans Fats Manufactured Artificially
The majority of trans fats in today's diet are derived from industrial hydrogenation of vegetable oils. To improve texture, shelf life, and flavor stability, this process is frequently used in the production of some

margarines, snack foods, fried foods, and baked goods. Certain margarines, baked goods, fried foods, and some snack foods are common sources.

Weight Gain

Trans fats are strongly linked to weight gain and obesity. They, like saturated fats, contribute to the caloric density of foods, and their excessive consumption can lead to an imbalance in energy intake. Trans fats can contribute to obesity by interfering with the metabolic processes of the body. They not only raise bad cholesterol but also lower good cholesterol, causing weight gain and increasing the risk of obesity-related diseases. Furthermore, trans fats may impair insulin sensitivity, potentially leading to increased fat storage and obesity.

Health Impact

Trans fats are especially harmful to cardiovascular health. They raise LDL (low-density lipoprotein) cholesterol levels while decreasing HDL (high-density lipoprotein) cholesterol levels. This unfavorable cholesterol profile raises the risk of cardiovascular disease, stroke, and other problems.

Recommendations

Trans fat consumption should be limited, according to all health guidelines. This can be accomplished by reading food labels for products containing partially hydrogenated oils and selecting alternatives with healthier fat profiles.

Fat That Helps You Lose Weight
Monounsaturated Fats

Monounsaturated fats are a type of dietary fat that, when consumed in moderation, is considered heart-healthy. These fats are known for their potential cardiovascular health benefits and are part of a well-balanced diet.

Primary Sources

Found in a variety of plant-based oils and foods.

Olive oil, avocados, nuts (such as almonds, peanuts, and cashews), and seeds (such as sesame seeds and pumpkin seeds) are good sources.

Chemical Structure

Monounsaturated fats have one double bond in their fatty acid chain.

Health Advantages

Heart Health

Monounsaturated fats have been linked to cardiovascular benefits such as improved lipid profiles. They can help lower LDL (low-density lipoprotein, or "bad" cholesterol) levels while maintaining or increasing HDL (high-density lipoprotein, or "good" cholesterol).

Inflammation

The anti-inflammatory properties of these fats contribute to overall cardiovascular health.

Sensitivity to Insulin

Monounsaturated fat consumption may improve insulin sensitivity, potentially lowering the risk of type 2 diabetes.

Satiety in weight management

Including monounsaturated fats in meals can increase satiety, potentially lowering overall calorie intake.

According to some research, diets high in monounsaturated fats may be more effective for weight loss than low-fat diets.

The Mediterranean Diet and Olive Oil

Olive oil is a key component of the Mediterranean diet, which has been linked to a variety of health benefits, including a lower risk of heart disease and certain cancers.

Olive Oil Extra Virgin

Extra virgin olive oil, considered the healthiest type of olive oil, retains more of the natural compounds found in olives, including antioxidants.

Including Monounsaturated Fats in Your Diet

Cooking

Cooking, sautéing, and salad dressing can all be done with olive oil.

Snacking

Snack on nuts and seeds for a healthy dose of monounsaturated fats.

Avocado Substitutions

Avocados can be used in salads, sandwiches, or as a topping for a variety of dishes.

Dietary Pattern in the Mediterranean Diet

The Mediterranean diet, which is high in monounsaturated fats, has been linked to lower rates of obesity, heart disease, and other chronic diseases.

Considerations

Whole Foods

This eating plan prioritizes wholesome, nutrient-rich foods like fruits, veggies, whole grains, lean proteins, and good fats, aiming for a well-rounded and healthy diet.

The Caloric Density

While monounsaturated fats have health benefits, they are high in calories. Moderation is essential, especially for those attempting to manage or lose weight.

Dietary Harmony

For a well-rounded diet, combine monounsaturated fats with a balanced intake of other healthy fats (polyunsaturated fats and omega-3 fatty acids), proteins, and carbohydrates.

Polyunsaturated fatty acids

Polyunsaturated fats are considered healthy fats that can be included in a balanced diet and may help with weight loss. These fats have a variety of health benefits and are well-known for their beneficial effects on heart health.

Polyunsaturated Fats and the Composition of a Lean Body
Multiple double bonds characterize the chemical structure. Polyunsaturated fats are distinguished from monounsaturated and saturated fats by the presence of multiple double bonds in their fatty acid chains.

Types of Polyunsaturated Fats

Fatty fish like salmon, mackerel, and sardines, along with flaxseeds, chia seeds, and walnuts, are sources of Omega-3 Fatty Acids, known for their anti-inflammatory properties.

Health Advantages

Heart Health

Omega-3 fatty acids, in particular, have been linked to cardiovascular benefits such as a lower risk of heart disease and higher cholesterol levels.

Brain Function

Essential for the health of the brain and cognitive function.

Inflammation

Polyunsaturated fats may have anti-inflammatory properties that benefit overall health.

Increased Metabolic Rate

According to some research, polyunsaturated fats may play a role in boosting metabolism, potentially aiding in weight management and a leaner body composition.

Energy Expenditure

Omega-3 fatty acids have been linked to increased fat-burning during exercise, which contributes to overall energy expenditure.

Appetite Control

Including polyunsaturated fats in meals may increase fullness and satisfaction, potentially lowering overall calorie intake.

Weight Loss
Some studies suggest that diets high in polyunsaturated fats can help you lose weight.

Examples of polyunsaturated fats
Fatty Fish
Consume salmon, mackerel, and sardines.
Flaxseeds and Chia Seeds
Sprinkle on yogurt or blend into smoothies.
Snack on nuts and seeds such as walnuts, flaxseeds, and chia seeds.
Plant Oils
Flaxseed oil and walnut oil can be used in salad dressings.

Considerations for Individuals

Genetic Factors

Genetic factors can influence how people react to dietary fats.

Health conditions

Individuals with certain health conditions, such as cardiovascular disease, may benefit from consuming more omega-3 fatty acids.

Omega-3 Essential Fatty Acids

Omega-3 fatty acids, a type of polyunsaturated fat, are frequently linked to a variety of health benefits, including a possible role in promoting a leaner body composition.

Examples of Omega-3 fatty acids
Fatty fish, such as salmon, mackerel, sardines, and trout, are high in omega-3 fatty acids.
 Fruits and seeds
Alpha-linolenic acid (ALA), a type of omega-3, is abundant in flaxseeds, chia seeds, walnuts, and hemp seeds.

Benefits of Omega-3 fatty acids

Enhanced Fat Burning

Omega-3 fatty acids, particularly EPA and DHA, have been linked to increased fat burning during exercise.

This can lead to increased energy expenditure and may aid in weight management.

Appetite Control

Omega-3 fatty acids may affect appetite regulation, assisting in the control of hunger and the prevention of overeating.

Feeling satisfied after meals can help with weight management.

Reduced fat storage

Some research suggests that omega-3 fatty acids may reduce fat storage in adipose tissue, potentially influencing body fat distribution.

This effect may help to achieve a leaner body composition.

Anti-Inflammatory Properties

Omega-3 fatty acids are widely recognized for their ability to reduce inflammation. Obesity is associated with chronic inflammation, and reducing inflammation may benefit overall metabolic health.

Improved insulin Sensitivity

Omega-3 fatty acids have been linked to increased insulin sensitivity.

Increased insulin sensitivity can help regulate blood sugar levels and may aid in weight loss.

Muscle Mass Preservation

Omega-3 fatty acids may help to increase muscle protein synthesis while decreasing muscle protein breakdown.

Maintaining lean muscle mass is critical for maintaining a healthy body composition. Omega-3 fatty acids have been linked to improved exercise performance and recovery.

Regular physical activity is essential for maintaining a healthy lifestyle.

Balancing Omega-3 to Omega-6 Fatty Acid

It is critical to maintain a healthy omega-3 to omega-6 fatty acid ratio.

Western diets are frequently imbalanced, with an excess of omega-6 fatty acids relative to omega-3s. Body composition can be improved by achieving balance.

Considerations for Supplementation
There are omega-3 supplements available, such as fish oil capsules. However, before beginning any supplementation, it is critical to consult with a healthcare professional.

Chapter 5

Putting together a diet to lose weight structurally.

Creating a diet plan with a balanced approach is necessary to lose weight. Prioritize lean proteins, emphasize portion control, include whole foods, and include a range of fruits and vegetables. Gaining structural weight loss requires an understanding of fundamental concepts. Start by managing your calories: eat fewer calories than your body uses.

Calorie control is essential for maintaining a healthy weight. It entails striking a balance between the number of calories your body uses for regular activities and metabolic processes and the number of calories you take in from food and drink. Create a calorie deficit by consuming fewer calories than your body requires to lose weight. Determine how many calories you need each day based on your age, gender, weight, degree of activity, and objectives. Reducing daily intake by 500–1,000 calories is a common strategy for losing weight gradually and sustainably, 1-2 pounds per week.

Putting into practice sensible weight-management and calorie-control techniques can help curb the obesity epidemic at the national level. To achieve it, follow these steps:

Equilibrium Energy
Controlling one's caloric intake makes sure that people eat in proportion to how much energy they use. This addresses one of the main causes of obesity by preventing the storage of excess energy as body fat.

Modifications in Behavior
Long-lasting behavioral changes are fostered by promoting portion control and healthier eating practices. This can eventually result in a decrease in

total caloric intake, which can help with weight loss and the prevention of obesity.

Metabolic Health

Nutrient intake balance promotes metabolic health by affecting variables such as insulin sensitivity. Enhancing metabolic function can help control weight and lower the chance of obesity-related diseases like type 2 diabetes.

Decreased Fat Cell Mass

Calorie control lowers the risk of obesity-related health problems by reducing excess adipose tissue. This is especially crucial because visceral fat is linked to disruptions in metabolism.

Modifications to Lifestyle

Encouraging regular physical activity improves general health and helps manage weight by working in tandem with calorie control. Leading an active lifestyle helps prevent and reduce obesity.

How Not to Cycle Your Weight

Calorie restriction aids in sustainable weight loss by breaking the cycle of weight gain and loss, which can be harmful to metabolic health. Retaining a steady weight lowers the likelihood of complications associated with obesity.

Insulin Resistance Prevention

Overeating can exacerbate insulin resistance, which is a condition associated with obesity. Refined sugars and fats are particularly high in insulin resistance. A balanced diet and calorie control help control blood sugar levels and lower the risk of insulin-related diseases.

Accept whole foods that promote satiety and are high in fiber, vitamins, and minerals. Minimize refined carbohydrates, sugary snacks, and processed foods. Hydration can reduce false hunger signals and speed up metabolism.

Adopting whole, high-fiber foods is the foundation of a nutritious diet and has many advantages.

Contentment and Control of Weight
Whole grains, fruits, and vegetables are examples of foods high in fiber that give you a feeling of fullness and satisfaction. Managing weight is facilitated by reducing overall caloric intake.

Health of the Digestive System
Fiber helps prevent constipation and promotes regular bowel movements. Additionally, it promotes the growth of good bacteria that are essential for digestion and general gut health,

maintaining a balanced gut microbiome.

The Impact of Gut Microbiota

As a prebiotic, fiber encourages the development of good gut flora. A more diverse and well-balanced gut microbiota has been linked to better metabolic health and a lower chance of obesity.

Blood Sugar Regulation

Foods high in soluble fiber, such as fruits, beans, and oats, can help control blood sugar levels. This is especially crucial for the management and prevention of diseases like type 2 diabetes.

Cardiovascular Health

Low cholesterol is linked to a diet high in fiber, particularly soluble fiber. Promoting heart health, in turn, lowers the risk of cardiovascular disorders.

Density of Nutrients

High-fiber whole foods are frequently teeming with vital elements, such as minerals, vitamins, and antioxidants. This encourages general well-being and gives the body the components it needs to perform at its best.

Maintaining Weight Loss Over Time

Encouraging good eating practices, including fiber in your diet will help you lose weight in a long-lasting way.

Foods high in fiber provide fewer calories per serving, so you can eat more of them without going overboard.

Control of Blood Pressure

Certain fiber sources, such as fruits and vegetables high in potassium, can help control blood pressure. For the sake of cardiovascular health, blood pressure regulation is essential.

Prevention of Diseases

A high-fiber diet has been linked to a decreased risk of several chronic illnesses, including some forms of cancer. The combination of nutrients and antioxidants present in whole, high-fiber diets may be the cause of the beneficial benefits.

Frequent Exercise

Frequent exercise improves calorie burning and advances general health by combining cardiovascular and strength training activities. Maintaining weight reduction over time requires consistency; it's a slow process.

Frequent exercise reduces and prevents obesity through several methods, including:

Energy Consumption

Your body burns more calories when you're moving about. When paired with a healthy diet, this caloric expenditure helps create a calorie deficit that promotes weight reduction and prevents obesity.

Rate of Metabolic Process

Exercise increases metabolism, both during and after the exercise. Because of this higher metabolic rate, your body burns calories long after you stop exercising, which helps you maintain a healthy weight.

Development of Muscle

Regular exercise encourages the growth of lean muscle mass, particularly strength training. An elevated basal metabolic rate is a result of muscle tissue burning more calories at rest than fat tissue.

Enhanced Sensitivity to Insulin

Exercise helps control blood sugar levels by increasing the body's sensitivity to insulin. This can be especially helpful in controlling and avoiding diseases like type 2 diabetes and insulin resistance, which are frequently linked to obesity.

Control of Appetite

Hormones involved in controlling hunger can be influenced by physical exercise. Exercise and hunger have a complicated relationship, but some research indicates that regular exercise may help manage desires and stop overeating.

Changes in Lifestyle

Regular exercise frequently results in more significant lifestyle adjustments. Regular exercisers are more likely to eat healthfully, which helps them maintain a healthy weight and avoid obesity.

Advantages of Exercise

Exercise improves mental health by lowering stress, anxiety, and depressive symptoms. Healthy eating habits and lifestyle decisions are associated with emotional well-being and can affect weight.

Sustaining Your Weight Loss

It is essential to engage in regular physical exercise to sustain weight loss. Encouraging long-term commitment to a healthy lifestyle and maintaining a maintained calorie balance, helps prevent the recovery of lost weight.

While exercise is an important component in the fight against obesity, it is most effective when accompanied by a well-balanced and healthy diet. Individual reactions to exercise might also differ, so consulting with healthcare specialists or fitness experts can give individualized advice for obtaining and maintaining a healthy weight.

Chapter 6

The Obesity Reduction Diet

The phrase "obesity fix diet" does not relate to a specific, widely accepted eating plan. Instead, it often refers to following a set of dietary guidelines and making lifestyle modifications to address and avoid obesity.

While there is no one-size-fits-all "obesity fix" diet, certain factors can contribute to a healthy and sustainable weight control strategy.

Individual requirements vary, thus seeking tailored advice from a healthcare expert or a qualified dietician is recommended. Following are some general guidelines:

Well-Balanced Diet

Emphasize a well-balanced diet rich in nutrient-dense foods. Include fruits, vegetables, whole grains, lean meats, and healthy fats to acquire a variety of critical elements.

Balance of Macronutrients
Proteins

Give priority to lean protein sources such as tofu, beans, fish, and poultry. Protein helps with weight reduction, increases satiety, and maintains muscle mass.

Glucose

Select complex carbs from fruits, vegetables, and whole grains. They support intestinal health and fullness by offering sustained energy and fiber.

Lipids

Choose healthy fats from nuts, avocados, and olive oil, among other sources. These fats aid in the absorption of nutrients and promote general health.

Calories Regulation

Establish a little calorie deficit to lose weight. This may be accomplished by consuming fewer calories overall, cutting back on portion sizes, and making lower-calorie food choices.

Strategies for Caloric Deficit

Portion Control

Pay attention to portion sizes to control total caloric intake. Controlling portions can be facilitated by using smaller dishes and being aware of signals of hunger and fullness.

Density of Nutrients

Choose nutrient-dense meals that are low in calories yet high in vitamins and minerals.

Foods High in Fiber

Incorporate high-fiber foods including legumes, whole grains, fruits, and vegetables. Fiber helps maintain healthy digestive tract function, blood sugar regulation, and satiety.

Options High in Fiber

Fruits and Vegetables

Eat more fruits and vegetables in your diet, both in terms of variety and quantity. These are high in fiber, antioxidants, and vitamins, which support general health and satiety.

Complete Grains

Select whole grains for more fiber and long-lasting energy, such as quinoa, brown rice, and oats.

Making selections high in fiber has the following advantages;

Encouraging Contentment

It's well known that fiber may make you feel satisfied and full. Foods high in fiber require more time to chew and digest, which can help regulate hunger and stop overindulging.

Regulation of Blood Sugar

Foods high in soluble fiber, such as fruits, legumes, and oats, can lower blood sugar levels by delaying the absorption of glucose. This may be especially helpful in reducing obesity-related disorders including type 2 diabetes and insulin resistance.

Gastrointestinal health

Whole grains and vegetables are rich sources of insoluble fiber, which helps maintain regular bowel motions by giving the stool more volume. This helps with gut health and can help with problems like constipation.

Lowering Density of Energy

When compared to meals with lower fiber content, foods high in fiber often have lower energy density, which means they deliver fewer calories for the same weight. This enables people to maintain calorie management while yet enjoying full servings.

Prolonged Weight Control

A diet rich in fiber is linked to effective long-term weight control. It facilitates the ingestion of foods that support general health, which makes it simpler to maintain long-term good eating practices.

Cut Back on Processed Foods and Added Sugars

Reduce your consumption of sweets, sugar-filled drinks, and highly processed meals. These frequently provide more calories while offering little nutritional benefit.

Cut Down on Empty Calories

"Empty" calories, or calories with no nutritional benefit, are what added sugars frequently supply. Reducing these empty calories is essential for a diet rich in nutrients and well-balanced.

Cut Down on Cravings

Processed meals, especially those heavy in sweets and bad fats, can activate the brain's reward regions, which can cause overindulgence and cravings. Restricting certain foods aids in controlling cravings and hunger.

Frequent Exercise

Sustain a well-rounded diet and participate in constant physical activity. Exercises that are aerobic (like jogging or walking) and strength-training enhance general health and assist with weight management.

Advantages of Regular Exercise

Caloric Consumption
Physical exercise increases the number of calories burned by your body, leading to a caloric deficit when paired with a healthy diet. This is necessary for weight management and can help with weight loss.

Increased Metabolism
Regular exercise, particularly strength training, can increase muscle mass and hence enhance metabolism. This implies that the body burns calories even when at rest, which aids in long-term weight maintenance.

Cardiovascular Wellness

Walking, jogging, swimming, and cycling are all aerobic workouts that promote cardiovascular health. They improve heart and lung function, lowering the risk of obesity-related cardiovascular disease.

Sensitivity to Insulin

Physical exercise promotes insulin sensitivity, which aids in blood sugar regulation. This is critical in avoiding and controlling obesity-related diseases such as insulin resistance and type 2 diabetes.

Appetite Control

Exercise can affect the hormones that regulate hunger. While the link is complicated, some research suggests that regular physical exercise may aid in the control of appetites and the prevention of overeating.

Improved Sleep Quality

Physical activity regularly can improve sleep quality, which is important for overall health and well-being. Weight gain and obesity are associated with insufficient sleep.

Water Intake

Ensure you stay well-hydrated by drinking a sufficient amount of water throughout the day. Hunger can sometimes be associated with dehydration. Drinking water before meals can help you feel fuller, potentially lowering your calorie intake and supporting your weight loss efforts.

Mindful Eating Techniques

Enhance your eating experience by engaging in mindful practices, and concentrating on the sensory aspects of your food. This reduces overeating and promotes a healthier relationship with food.

Mindful eating is a method of eating that encourages heightened awareness and intentional focus on the present moment. It entails paying attention to the sensory aspects of eating and cultivating a stronger bond between mind and body. Here's a closer examination of these principles:

Focus on the Present

Reduce distractions such as phones or television when having a meal. Enhance your eating experience by engaging in mindful practices, and concentrating on the sensory aspects of your food.

Pay Attention to Hunger Signs

Take note of your body's hunger cues. Consume food in response to physical hunger, rather than during periods of boredom or emotional stress.

Recognize Completeness

Keep an eye out for sensations that indicate fullness. Even if there is food left over, stop eating when you are satisfied.

Mind-Body Relationship

Slow down your eating pace to allow your body to register fullness. Take your time with each bite, savoring the flavors and textures.

Recognize Emotional Triggers

Recognize emotional eating triggers such as stress, boredom, or sadness. Separating these emotions from eating encourages a healthier relationship with food.

Portion Control

Use mindful practices to determine proper portion sizes. Pay attention to your body's signals of satisfaction to avoid overeating.

Avoid self-criticism

Approach your eating habits with compassion and without judgment. Be mindful of any negative self-talk about food choices.

Intentional Eating

Make deliberate decisions about what and how much you eat. Consider the nutritional value of your food and select options that will benefit your health.

Behavioral Reinforcement

Practicing good practices regularly promotes beneficial behaviors. These actions become routine over time, making it easier to sustain a healthy lifestyle.

Patience and consistency

It takes time to achieve long-term weight loss. Maintain your healthy behaviors and prioritize gradual, long-term changes over fast cures.

Adopting and keeping healthy behaviors requires consistency and patience, especially when it comes to treating issues such as obesity. Here's a more in-depth look at these principles:

Continual Practice

Committing to consistently practicing good activities is what consistency entails. This involves eating a well-balanced diet, getting enough exercise, and making other healthy lifestyle adjustments.

Creating Routines

Creating consistent routines aids in the formation of habits that get established in daily life. Consistency supports healthy behaviors, whether it's meal planning, workout regimens, or sleeping patterns.

Gradual Advancement

Consistency may not always necessitate radical adjustments. Small, persistent improvements over time can lead to great progress and long-term success.

Behavioral Reinforcement

Practicing good practices regularly promotes beneficial behaviors. These actions become routine over time, making it easier to sustain a healthy lifestyle.

Adaptability

Perfection does not imply consistency. It entails a continuous effort to make healthy choices while realizing that deviations or setbacks are a typical part of the journey.

Patience
Realistic Expectations

Setting realistic progress expectations requires patience. Healthy, long-term improvements take time, and expecting rapid benefits can lead to disappointment.

Long-Term Perspective

Patience entails taking a long-term view of one's health and well-being. Rather than seeking quick fixes, concentrate on incremental, long-term changes that contribute to long-term benefits.

Mindful Progress Tracking

Rather than focusing on the scale or short-term results, exercise patience by focusing on total well-being. Keep track of your energy levels, mood, and overall health.

Acknowledge and Celebrate Tiny Accomplishments

Patience is maintained by acknowledging progress, even if it is not always obvious.

Learning from Setbacks

Patience entails accepting that setbacks are an inevitable part of any path. Instead of being a source of despair, view failures as chances for learning and progress.

In conclusion, consistency and patience are critical components of a successful and long-term approach to combating obesity and boosting general well-being. Accepting incremental development, making consistent efforts, and cultivating resilience all contribute to a beneficial and long-term impact on one's health.